Sacroiliac Joint Pain Diet

A Beginner's 3-Step Plan to Managing Joint Dysfunction Through Diet, with Sample Recipes and a Meal Plan

mf

copyright © 2022 Tyler Spellmann

All rights reserved No part of this book may be reproduced, or stored in a retrieval system, or transmitted in any form or by any means, electronic, mechanical, photocopying, recording, or otherwise, without express written permission of the publisher.

Disclaimer

By reading this disclaimer, you are accepting the terms of the disclaimer in full. If you disagree with this disclaimer, please do not read the guide.

All of the content within this guide is provided for informational and educational purposes only, and should not be accepted as independent medical or other professional advice. The author is not a doctor, physician, nurse, mental health provider, or registered nutritionist/dietician. Therefore, using and reading this guide does not establish any form of a physician-patient relationship.

Always consult with a physician or another qualified health provider with any issues or questions you might have regarding any sort of medical condition. Do not ever disregard any qualified professional medical advice or delay seeking that advice because of anything you have read in this guide. The information in this guide is not intended to be any sort of medical advice and should not be used in lieu of any medical advice by a licensed and qualified medical professional.

The information in this guide has been compiled from a variety of known sources. However, the author cannot attest to or guarantee the accuracy of each source and thus should not be held liable for any errors or omissions.

You acknowledge that the publisher of this guide will not be held liable for any loss or damage of any kind incurred as a result of this guide or the reliance on any information provided within this guide. You acknowledge and agree that you assume all risk and responsibility for any action you undertake in response to the information in this guide.

Using this guide does not guarantee any particular result (e.g., weight loss or a cure). By reading this guide, you acknowledge that there are no guarantees to any specific outcome or results you can expect.

All product names, diet plans, or names used in this guide are for identification purposes only and are the property of their respective owners. The use of these names does not imply endorsement. All other trademarks cited herein are the property of their respective owners.

Where applicable, this guide is not intended to be a substitute for the original work of this diet plan and is, at most, a supplement to the original work for this diet plan and never a direct substitute. This guide is a personal expression of the facts of that diet plan.

Where applicable, persons shown in the cover images are stock photography models and the publisher has obtained the rights to use the images through license agreements with third-party stock image companies.

Table of Contents

Introduction   7
All About Sacroiliac Joint Pain   9
    Causes   10
    Risk Factors   11
    Symptoms of Sacroiliitis   13
    About Sacroiliitis   13
    Diagnosis of Sacroiliac Joint Dysfunction   14
    Treatment   15
Managing Sacroiliac Joint Pain   17
    Avoid high-impact activities   17
    Try SI joints-safe exercises   17
    Use heat and cold therapy   18
    Practice good posture   18
    Stretch and strengthen the muscles around the joints   19
    Use an SI joint brace or belt   19
    Lose excess weight   20
    Curate your diet   20
Healthy Lifestyle Helps   21
    Practicing good posture   21
    Staying active   22
Following a Healthy Diet for Sacroiliac Joint Pain   23
    Principles of the Anti-Inflammatory Diet for Sacroiliac Joint Disease   23
    Benefits of the Anti-Inflammatory Diet for Sacroiliac Joint Disease   25
    Potential Disadvantages of the Anti-Inflammatory Diet for Sacroiliac Joint Disease   27
The Three-Step Plan   30
    Step One: Create Your Meal Plans   30
    Step Two: Start Slowly   33

Step Three: Stay Active	36
Foods to Avoid for Sacroiliac Joint Pain	41
Foods to Eat	41
Sample Recipes	**44**
Apple and Onion Soup	45
Trout Scrambler	46
Grilled Halibut Niçoise with Mixed Vegetables	48
Salmon Fry	50
Kale Salad with Strawberry & Almonds	51
Tuna Salad	52
Orange-Walnut Salad	53
Strawberry, Blueberry, and Spinach Salad	54
Kale Fried Rice	56
Instant Pot Bone Broth	58
Garlic Hummus	60
Blueberry Pancakes with Whipped Cream	61
Energy Oats	63
Tomato and Basil Soup	64
Roasted Broccoli and Salmon	66
Tuna and Veggies Wrap	68
Barley and Chicken Soup	69
Garlic-Cashews Red Pasta	71
Exotic Empanadas	72
Pork Tenderloin	74
Baked Turkey Wings	75
Conclusion	**76**
FAQs for Sacroiliac Joint Disease Management Through Diet 80	
References and Helpful Links	**83**

Introduction

Sacroiliac Joint Disease (SIJD) is a condition that affects many people, causing considerable discomfort and often disrupting daily activities. Research indicates that 10-25% of back pain experienced by adults can be attributed to sacroiliac joints. This type of pain can be debilitating, primarily affecting the lower back and buttocks.

The pain from SIJD arises due to the breakdown of cartilage that cushions these joints, leading to bone-on-bone contact. This results in inflammation, stiffness, and significant discomfort. Typical treatments for sacroiliac joint pain include physical therapy, exercises, and medications. In severe cases, surgery may be required to address the issue. However, managing symptoms through diet is a practical and proactive approach that can complement other treatments.

Adopting a well-balanced and nutritious diet is a great starting point for those looking to manage their SIJD symptoms. Foods rich in omega-3 fatty acids, antioxidants, and essential vitamins can reduce inflammation and support joint health. By making informed dietary choices, individuals can take control of their condition and improve their overall health and well-being.

This beginner's guide offers a three-step plan to help individuals manage sacroiliitis through diet. It includes valuable insights into sacroiliac joint pain, its symptoms, and risk factors, as well as practical advice on starting the sacroiliac joint pain diet. The guide also provides sample recipes to make the transition easier.

By following the strategies outlined in this guide, individuals can embark on a journey towards reduced pain and enhanced quality of life. Here is what you will discover in this quick-start guide:

- Helpful information about sacroiliac joint pain
- Symptoms and risk factors of SI joint pain
- Strategies for managing the condition
- Steps to start the sacroiliac joint pain diet
- A three-step plan to work on the diet and sample recipes

With these practical tips and nutritious recipes, readers can easily incorporate these dietary changes into their daily routine, taking a significant step towards comfort and better joint health.

All About Sacroiliac Joint Pain

Sacroiliac joint pain or dysfunction is a condition that can cause pain in the lower back and buttocks. Approximately 1 in 4 people will experience sacroiliac joint pain at some point in their life. The cause of the pain is not always clear, but it is thought to be related to inflammation or injury of the sacroiliac joints.

The pain experienced in this area is also related to either excessive movement or hypermobility (instability) and lack of movement or hypomobility.

The sacroiliac (SI) joint is a joint that connects the sacrum—the triangular bone at the bottom of the spine—to the ilium, or the hip bone. The sacroiliac joints help to support the weight of the body and allow for movement in the hips and lower back. When these joints are damaged or inflamed, it can lead to pain and difficulty moving. This joint is often the source of pain in people who have chronic lower back pain.

Causes

Here are some common causes of SI joint dysfunction, as listed by the Weill Cornell Brain and Spine Center:

1. *Arthritis and Degenerative Joint Diseases*: These conditions can lead to the deterioration of the cartilage in the SI joints.
2. *Ankylosing Spondylitis*: A chronic inflammatory disease and type of arthritis that affects the lower back, potentially causing fusion of some spine bones.
3. *Injury*: Traumatic incidents such as falls or hard impacts to the buttocks can strain or tear the ligaments in the SI joints, leading to dysfunction.
4. *Pregnancy*: During pregnancy, the changes in a woman's body, including weight gain and preparation for childbirth, put extra stress on the SI joints, which may cause inflammation.
5. *Uneven Leg Length*: Individuals with legs of different lengths, due to conditions or accidents, experience uneven leg movement that stresses the SI joint, triggering pain.
6. *Post-Surgery Injury*: After foot or ankle surgery, failing to wear proper footwear when walking can lead to degenerative inflammatory sacroiliitis.

By understanding the potential causes of SI joint dysfunction, individuals can take steps to prevent or manage their symptoms through proper medical treatment and lifestyle adjustments. Depending on the underlying cause, treatments may include physical therapy, medication, corticosteroid injections, or surgery.

Risk Factors

Here are some risk factors that can increase the likelihood of developing sacroiliitis:

1. **Being Overweight or Obese**: Carrying excess weight puts additional stress on the sacroiliac (SI) joints, which can lead to increased pain and discomfort. This added pressure may exacerbate existing joint issues and contribute to the development of other related conditions.
2. **History of Back Pain**: Previous episodes of back pain, whether chronic or acute, can significantly contribute to the development of SI joint issues. This is often due to the stress and strain placed on the surrounding structures, which can lead to inflammation and instability over time.
3. **Scoliosis**: This condition involves an abnormal lateral curvature of the spine, which can significantly affect the alignment and function of the SI joints. Over time, the misalignment caused by scoliosis can lead to discomfort and mobility issues.
4. **Family History**: If you have a genetic predisposition, such as a history of certain conditions or diseases in

your family, this may increase your risk. It's important to be aware of your family's health background and discuss it with your healthcare provider.

5. *Autoimmune Disorders*: Conditions like rheumatoid arthritis can lead to inflammation of the SI joints, causing chronic pain and stiffness. This inflammation occurs when the immune system mistakenly attacks healthy tissues, resulting in discomfort and impaired joint function.

6. *Smoking Cigarettes*: Smoking is associated with various inflammatory conditions, including sacroiliitis. The harmful chemicals in cigarettes can contribute to inflammation and aggravate existing conditions, making it harder for the body to heal and increasing the risk of chronic pain.

7. *Jobs or Activities that Involve Repetitive Strain on the SI Joints*: Certain occupations or hobbies that involve frequent bending, heavy lifting, or twisting can put a strain on the SI joints and increase the risk of developing sacroiliitis.

8. *Pregnancy and Childbirth*: As mentioned earlier, pregnancy can cause changes in the pelvic area and extra stress on the SI joints, leading to inflammation.

9. *Sports Injuries*: Injuries sustained during high-impact sports such as football or soccer can damage the SI joints and potentially lead to sacroiliitis.

It's important to note that having one or more of these risk factors does not necessarily mean you will develop sacroiliitis. Many people with these risk factors may never experience any SI joint problems. However, it's important to be aware of them and take steps to prevent or manage the condition if needed.

Symptoms of Sacroiliitis

If you are experiencing any of the following symptoms, you may have sacroiliitis:

- *Lower Back and Hip Pain*: Pain that worsens after sitting for a long time or when getting up from a seated position.
- *Stiffness*: Stiffness in the lower back and hips.
- *Difficulty Walking or Standing*: Challenges in walking or standing up straight.
- *Locking Sensation*: Feeling like your hips or back are locking up or giving out on you.
- *Numbness or Tingling*: Sensations of numbness or tingling in the buttocks.

About Sacroiliitis

Sacroiliitis occurs when the sacroiliac (SI) joints are not functioning properly, leading to pain and inflammation in the surrounding area. Those with this condition often experience worsening pain during everyday activities such as climbing stairs, moving around in bed, and standing up or sitting down for extended periods. Running and standing on one leg can also exacerbate the pain.

Additional Symptoms of Sacroiliitis:

- Fever
- Pain in the Lower Back and Buttocks
- Stiffness and Difficulty Moving the Hips
- Swelling in the Joints
- Pain When Standing or Walking
- Pain That Increases When Sitting or Lying Down

Diagnosis of Sacroiliac Joint Dysfunction

To diagnose sacroiliac (SI) joint dysfunction, doctors may perform several tests to rule out other conditions, especially if the patient has a history of inflammatory disorders. These diagnostic tests may include:

- *Blood Tests*: These tests are conducted to detect any signs of inflammation in the body.
- *Imaging Tests*: Commonly known as X-rays, CT scans, and MRI scans, these tests help identify the source of pain or observe any changes in the SI joint.
- *Physical Exam*: During this exam, the alignment and rotation of the spine, including the hip, leg, and sacroiliac joint, are checked by applying pressure.

Increased pain during these movement tests may indicate SI dysfunction or sacroiliitis.
- *Steroid Injection*: This test not only helps diagnose but also treats SI joint pain. Steroids are injected into the SI joint using an X-ray for guidance. If relief is experienced after the injection, it confirms SI joint pain.

These diagnostic tests, along with detailed patient history and physical examination, help doctors accurately diagnose sacroiliitis.

Treatment

There are several treatment options available for people with sacroiliac joint dysfunction, including:

- *Resting*: Avoid activities that cause pain or discomfort, allowing your body time to heal and reduce inflammation.
- *Applying Ice or Heat*: Use cold compresses to reduce swelling and numbing pain or warm compresses to relax muscles and improve blood flow to the affected area.
- *Regular Exercise*: Engage in low-impact exercises that strengthen and stabilize the SI joints, such as yoga, pilates, or specific physical therapy exercises designed for joint health.

- ***Pain Medications***: Take over-the-counter pain relief medications, such as ibuprofen or acetaminophen, or consult your doctor for prescription options if the pain is severe.
- ***Physical Therapy or Chiropractic Care***: Consider professional treatments, including physical therapy exercises to improve strength and flexibility, or chiropractic adjustments to improve joint function and alignment.
- ***Dietary and Lifestyle Changes***: Adopt a healthy diet rich in anti-inflammatory foods, maintain a healthy weight to reduce joint stress, and incorporate lifestyle changes such as quitting smoking and reducing alcohol intake to support overall joint health.

With proper treatment and management, most people with sacroiliitis can experience significant relief from their symptoms. It is essential to work closely with a healthcare professional to determine the best treatment plan for each individual case.

Managing Sacroiliac Joint Pain

There are different ways to treat this condition, particularly in managing the pain. Aside from medications, there are also home remedies you can do to help manage the pain or even alleviate the symptoms.

Avoid high-impact activities

High-impact activities like running can aggravate sacroiliac joint pain. If you enjoy running or doing other high-impact activities, try to take it easy on your joints and be sure to warm up before starting. If possible, try doing low-impact activities or exercises instead, like walking. Just make sure you'll do some proper stretching before doing these activities.

Try SI joints-safe exercises

There are also other specific exercises, such as yoga, that help condition and strengthen the SI joints. Yoga poses like child's pose, cat-cow, and bridge pose can be particularly beneficial. Make sure though that you're able to handle these exercises by starting slowly and listening to your body.

If you feel any pain or discomfort, skip the exercise and find a better alternative that suits your condition. Including gentle stretching and low-impact activities can also be helpful. Better yet, consult with a therapist or a healthcare professional to tailor a safe and effective exercise plan for your individual needs.

Use heat and cold therapy

Applying heat or cold to the affected area can help relieve pain and reduce inflammation. Heat therapy, such as using a warm towel or heating pad, can help increase blood flow and relax tight muscles, making it particularly effective for chronic pain or stiffness. Cold therapy, like ice packs or cold compresses, can numb the affected area and reduce swelling, which is especially beneficial for acute injuries or inflammation.

Try alternating between hot and cold packs, or taking a warm bath to see what works best for you. Experiment with different durations and temperatures to find the most effective combination for your specific condition. Remember to always wrap heat and cold packs in a cloth to protect your skin and avoid prolonged exposure to prevent burns or frostbite.

Practice good posture

Maintaining good posture can help take the pressure off of your sacroiliac joints and reduce the risk of discomfort or injury. When sitting, stand tall with your shoulders back and down, ensuring your back is straight and supported.

Consider using a cushion or lumbar support if needed. When standing, keep your weight evenly balanced on both feet and avoid slouching by engaging your core muscles. Regularly check your posture throughout the day to make necessary adjustments.

Stretch and strengthen the muscles around the joints

Stretching and strengthening the muscles around the sacroiliac joints can help support the joints and reduce pain. Engaging in regular, gentle stretching exercises like yoga or Pilates can improve flexibility and muscle strength, which in turn provides better support to the joints. Additionally, consider working with a physical therapist to find specific exercises tailored to your condition.

A professional can guide you through a customized exercise plan that targets the areas needing the most attention, ensuring you get the most benefit with minimal risk of injury. Regular practice of these exercises can lead to significant improvements in joint stability and overall comfort.

Use an SI joint brace or belt

Braces and belts for SI joints are used to support and compress the joints, which restricts them from excessive movement. These also help lessen the pain. Doing so lessens the stress on the SI joints. This is perfect for those who are hypermobile or move around a lot. Take note though, that wearing SI joint braces or belts shouldn't be considered a long-term solution.

Lose excess weight

This is one of the more long-term remedies to deal with sacroiliac joint pain, however, its benefits are also long-term. When you gain weight, your bones—particularly the spine, and joints on the hips, pelvic, and sacroiliac—work harder to keep your body upright. When you lose excess weight, the stress on your body also eases up.

Curate your diet

To help you lose weight, it's good to follow a diet, which will also help alleviate the symptoms you're experiencing with your condition. One of the most important things you should do first is to consult with your doctor and a dietician regarding the best diet plan to follow or food items you need to consume more as well as the ones you need to remove from your diet.

Based on those food items, try to curate meal plans that will be beneficial for you and your health.

Healthy Lifestyle Helps

Choosing to live healthy will get anyone a long way. This is extremely beneficial, especially for people with conditions that affect them for most of their lives. It's important to take the medications prescribed by health professionals, but it's also encouraged that patients do things that aid in improving their symptoms, whether by following a strict diet, maintaining an active lifestyle, or following a routine or regimen that may be beneficial for their needs.

Practicing good posture

Everything great starts with something simple. One of the simplest yet effective ways to help cope with your condition is by practicing good posture and maintaining this until it becomes a part of you. If you think doing posture exercises helps you, then go ahead and try doing them and stick to them.

You can also invest in getting effective tools that aid in correcting posture, or better yet, go and see a posture therapist. You may also involve your family in this simple exercise by appointing each other as your accountability partner.

While this may not necessarily treat your SI joint pain, this type of simple exercise will help lessen the burden you may feel from your condition, which will eventually benefit you in the long run.

Staying active

Maintaining an active lifestyle without adding too much strain to your sacroiliac joints may benefit you greatly. Because you still have to move around, it is only logical that you try to find ways to help strengthen your body.

Just as mentioned in the previous chapter, there are different stretching and strengthening exercises that you can do to help your body as well as to try to lessen the symptoms.

Make sure that you ask your doctor about these types of exercises before actually doing them. It's best if they could recommend either exercises you can do or a trainer or therapist to help you with exercise routines that will be beneficial for you.

Following a Healthy Diet for Sacroiliac Joint Pain

A healthy diet provides numerous benefits for individuals with sacroiliac (SI) joint pain. Nutrient-rich foods, including vitamins, minerals, and antioxidants, can help reduce inflammation and improve joint health. Additionally, maintaining a healthy weight through proper nutrition can reduce stress on the joints.

Principles of the Anti-Inflammatory Diet for Sacroiliac Joint Disease

1. **Focus on Whole Foods**
- Emphasize fresh fruits, vegetables, whole grains, lean proteins, and healthy fats.
- Aim to minimize processed foods and refined sugars.
2. **Incorporate Omega-3 Fatty Acids**
- Include sources like fatty fish (salmon, mackerel, sardines), flaxseeds, chia seeds, and walnuts.
- Omega-3s are known for their anti-inflammatory properties.

3. **Increase Antioxidant Intake**
   - Consume a variety of colorful fruits and vegetables such as berries, leafy greens, and bell peppers.
   - Antioxidants combat oxidative stress and inflammation.
4. **Limit Pro-Inflammatory Foods**
   - Reduce intake of foods high in saturated fats, trans fats, and sugar.
   - Avoid processed meats, fried foods, and sugary beverages.
5. **Opt for Whole Grains**
   - Replace refined grains with whole grains like brown rice, quinoa, and whole oats.
   - Whole grains have more fiber and nutrients that support inflammation reduction.
6. **Choose Healthy Fats**
   - Use olive oil, avocado oil, and nuts as primary fat sources.
   - Avoid unhealthy fats found in fast food and commercially baked goods.
7. **Stay Hydrated**
   - Drink plenty of water throughout the day.
   - Proper hydration helps maintain joint health and overall body function.
8. **Limit Dairy and Red Meat**
   - Some individuals find relief by reducing dairy and red meat consumption.

- Opt for plant-based proteins or lean meats like poultry and fish.

9. **Spice it Up**
- Incorporate anti-inflammatory spices like turmeric, ginger, garlic, and cinnamon into meals.
- These spices have natural anti-inflammatory properties.

10. **Moderate Alcohol Consumption**
- Limit alcohol intake as excessive drinking can promote inflammation.
- If consumed, opt for red wine in moderation due to its potential anti-inflammatory benefits.

11. **Maintain a Balanced Diet**
- Aim for a variety of nutrients to support overall health.
- Balance macronutrients (carbohydrates, proteins, fats) appropriately.

Following these principles can help manage inflammation and potentially alleviate symptoms associated with Sacroiliac Joint Disease. Always consult with a healthcare provider before making significant dietary changes.

Bencfits of the Anti-Inflammatory Diet for Sacroiliac Joint Disease

Incorporating an anti-inflammatory diet into your lifestyle can provide numerous benefits for those living with Sacroiliac

Joint Disease. Here are some potential advantages of following this approach:

1. **Reduced Inflammation**: The primary benefit is the reduction of inflammation in the sacroiliac joints, leading to decreased pain and discomfort.
2. **Improved Joint Function**: By reducing inflammation, the diet can help improve joint mobility and overall function, making daily activities easier to perform.
3. **Pain Relief**: Many individuals experience significant pain relief as inflammation decreases, which can enhance quality of life.
4. **Enhanced Healing**: A nutrient-rich diet supports the body's natural healing processes, promoting quicker recovery from flare-ups and injuries.
5. **Weight Management**: This diet often leads to healthier body weight by focusing on whole, nutrient-dense foods, which can reduce stress on the sacroiliac joints.
6. **Better Digestive Health**: High-fiber foods included in the diet promote good digestive health, which can contribute to overall well-being and reduce systemic inflammation.
7. **Increased Energy Levels**: A balanced, anti-inflammatory diet can increase energy levels by providing steady, sustained sources of nutrition.
8. **Lower Risk of Comorbidities**: Reducing inflammation can lower the risk of developing other chronic

conditions such as heart disease, diabetes, and other inflammatory diseases.
9. ***Enhanced Immune Function***: Nutrient-dense foods support a stronger immune system, helping the body fight off infections and illnesses that could exacerbate joint issues.
10. ***Balanced Blood Sugar Levels***: The diet helps maintain stable blood sugar levels, reducing spikes that can contribute to inflammation.
11. ***Decreased Dependency on Medications***: With reduced inflammation and pain, there may be a decreased need for anti-inflammatory medications or painkillers, lowering the risk of side effects.
12. ***Improved Mental Health***: Chronic pain and inflammation can affect mental health; reducing these symptoms can lead to better mood and overall mental well-being.

Overall, an anti-inflammatory diet offers a holistic approach to managing Sacroiliac Joint Disease, addressing both the symptoms and underlying causes.

Potential Disadvantages of the Anti-Inflammatory Diet for Sacroiliac Joint Disease

While there are many potential benefits to following an anti-inflammatory diet for Sacroiliac Joint Disease, it may not be suitable for everyone. Here are some factors to consider before adopting this dietary approach:

1. **Dietary Restrictions and Compliance**: Adhering to an anti-inflammatory diet often requires significant lifestyle changes, which can be challenging for many individuals. The need to consistently avoid certain foods that contribute to inflammation, such as processed foods, sugary beverages, and red meats, might feel restrictive and hard to maintain over the long term.
2. **Nutritional Deficiencies**: Although anti-inflammatory diets are generally well-balanced, there's a potential risk of nutritional deficiencies if not carefully planned. For instance, avoiding dairy or certain grains without suitable replacements could lead to a lack of essential nutrients like calcium or fiber.
3. **Cost and Accessibility Anti-inflammatory**: diets often emphasize the consumption of fresh fruits, vegetables, whole grains, and healthy fats, which can sometimes be more expensive and less accessible than processed alternatives. This can pose a financial burden or accessibility issue for some individuals.

Despite these challenges, the benefits of an anti-inflammatory diet, including reduced joint inflammation and overall improved health, typically outweigh the disadvantages. By mitigating inflammation through diet, individuals may experience significant relief from symptoms associated with Sacroiliac Joint Disease and better long-term health outcomes.

The Three-Step Plan

Now that you have a basic understanding of how a healthy diet can help to reduce sacroiliac joint pain, let's get started on your three-step plan.

Step One: Create Your Meal Plans

For starters, it's always best to begin a new program by planning your meals. This way, you'll be able to get into the program little by little, slowly removing the food items from your pantry that you need to avoid and replacing them with better, highly recommended alternatives.

As we discussed in the previous chapter, there are a few key nutrients that are especially important for people with sacroiliac (SI) joint pain: vitamin D, omega-3 fatty acids, and vitamin C. Make sure you include plenty of foods that are rich in these nutrients in your diet.

Key Nutrient Sources:

Vitamin D

- Fatty fish, such as salmon, tuna, and mackerel

- Eggs
- Fortified milk

Omega-3 Fatty Acids

- Fatty fish, such as salmon, tuna, and mackerel
- Plant-based oils, such as flaxseed oil and chia seed oil

Vitamin C

- Citrus fruits, such as oranges and grapefruits
- Strawberries
- Bell peppers
- Brussels sprouts
- Broccoli

In addition to getting enough of these key nutrients, you should also make sure you're eating plenty of fruits and vegetables. Fruits and vegetables are packed with antioxidants, vitamins, minerals, and fiber. They are also low in calories and unhealthy fats. Eating plenty of fruits and vegetables can help to reduce inflammation and provide the nutrients needed for healthy joints.

Start by planning your meals for an entire week. Plot your meals per day. This will help you make sure that you get the right nutrients for your daily needs. Once you have listed down your preferred meals for the day, do your grocery at the start of the week.

Below is a sample 7-day meal plan you can use as a guide:

Sample 7-Day Meal Plan

Day 1

- Breakfast: Blueberry Pancakes with Whipped Cream
- Lunch: Salmon Fry
- Dinner: Apple and Onion Soup

Day 2

- Breakfast: Kale Salad with Strawberry & Almonds
- Lunch: Trout Scrambler
- Dinner: Tuna and Veggies Wrap

Day 3

- Breakfast: Tuna Salad
- Lunch: Grilled Halibut Niçoise with Mixed Vegetables
- Dinner: Pork Tenderloin

Day 4

- Breakfast: Orange-Walnut Salad
- Lunch: Garlic-Cashews Red Pasta
- Dinner: Instant Pot Bone Broth

Day 5

- Breakfast: Strawberry, Blueberry, and Spinach Salad
- Lunch: Tomato and Basil Soup
- Dinner: Roasted Broccoli and Salmon

Day 6

- Breakfast: Energy Oats
- Lunch: Kale Fried Rice
- Dinner: Baked Turkey Wings

Day 7

- Breakfast: Garlic Hummus
- Lunch: Barley and Chicken Soup
- Dinner: Exotic Empanadas

By following this meal plan and incorporating the suggested nutrient-rich foods, you'll be on your way to reducing inflammation and supporting healthy joints.

Step Two: Start Slowly

In case you're not used to eating healthy, one way to make this journey enjoyable and still successful is by starting slowly. This gradual approach ensures that the transition into an anti-inflammatory diet is sustainable and not overwhelming. Here are some effective strategies to help you ease into this new lifestyle:

Substitute One Meal at a Time

Begin by substituting one meal with a strict anti-inflammatory meal at least three times a week. For instance, you could start with breakfast on Mondays, Wednesdays, and Fridays. Choose meals rich in anti-inflammatory foods such as berries, nuts, and whole grains.

Berries like blueberries and strawberries are packed with antioxidants that fight inflammation, while nuts like almonds and walnuts provide healthy fats and protein. Whole grains like oats and quinoa offer fiber and nutrients.

As you become more comfortable with these changes, gradually increase the frequency of these substitutions. After a few weeks, aim to incorporate an anti-inflammatory meal once a day. Eventually, you can transition into eating healthier meals twice a day, and finally, fully commit to the anti-inflammatory program.

For example, you might start having a nutritious lunch or dinner that includes vegetables like spinach and kale, lean proteins like salmon or tofu, and anti-inflammatory spices such as turmeric and ginger.

This methodical progression helps your body and taste buds adjust without feeling deprived or overwhelmed. It prevents the transition from feeling like a fad diet, which often leads to quick burnout.

Instead, it fosters a long-term commitment to healthier eating habits. By taking gradual steps, you allow yourself to experiment and find new recipes and foods that you enjoy, making the journey to better health more sustainable and enjoyable. Remember, the goal is to make lasting changes that support your overall well-being, rather than temporary fixes that are hard to maintain.

Keep a Food Diary

Another way to assist you in transitioning slowly is by making a food diary. Using a food diary will help you track not only the food recipes you have already tried but also how you feel about them. Record details such as ingredients, preparation methods, and your personal reactions to each meal. Note any improvements in your symptoms, energy levels, and overall well-being.

This practice offers several benefits:

- *Personalized Insights*: Understand which foods work best for you and which ones may not suit your palate or nutritional needs.
- *Identifying Patterns*: Recognize any patterns between your diet and how you feel, helping to make informed decisions about future meals.
- *Staying Accountable*: Maintaining a food diary encourages accountability and consistency in following the diet.
- *Meal Planning*: Use the diary to curate future meal plans, ensuring they include your favorite recipes and variations that you enjoy.

For example, if you noticed that you particularly enjoyed a kale and berry smoothie for breakfast and felt energized afterward, you might choose to incorporate that recipe more frequently. Conversely, if a certain recipe doesn't appeal to you, you can avoid it in the future, making your diet both effective and enjoyable.

Explore New Recipes

Explore new and exciting recipes that align with the anti-inflammatory diet. Experimenting with different cuisines and cooking methods can keep your meals interesting and prevent monotony. Incorporate a variety of fruits, vegetables, whole grains, lean proteins, and healthy fats to ensure a balanced and flavorful diet.

By starting slowly and embracing these strategies, you'll create a positive and lasting relationship with healthy eating. This gradual approach not only makes the transition smoother but also increases the likelihood of sticking to the diet in the long term, ultimately leading to significant health benefits.

Step Three: Stay Active

Exercise is an essential component of a healthy lifestyle. It can help reduce weight, improve joint function, and increase muscle strength, all of which can contribute to reducing sacroiliac (SI) joint pain. Regular physical activity not only supports your physical health but also enhances mental well-being, providing a holistic approach to managing SI joint pain.

The Benefits of Exercise for SI Joint Pain

- *Weight Reduction*: Excess body weight can add stress to the SI joints, exacerbating pain. Engaging in regular exercise helps manage weight, thereby reducing the pressure on these joints.
- *Improved Joint Function*: Movement helps lubricate the joints, keeping them flexible and functional. Exercise promotes circulation and the delivery of nutrients to the joints.
- *Increased Muscle Strength*: Strengthening the muscles around the SI joint provides better support and stability, reducing the likelihood of pain and injury.

Starting Slowly

If you're not used to exercising, it's crucial to start off slowly. Jumping into an intense exercise regimen too quickly can lead to injuries and discourage continued participation. Here are some steps to help you ease into a regular exercise routine:

1. **Consult Your Doctor:**

   Before beginning any new exercise program, especially if you have existing health conditions or chronic pain, consult with your doctor. They can provide guidance tailored to your specific needs and limitations. Additionally, your doctor may suggest specific exercises or modifications to ensure you exercise safely and effectively. This step is crucial to prevent injury and to make sure your fitness journey aligns with your overall health plan.

2. **Begin with Basic Exercises:**

Start with low-impact exercises that are gentle on the joints. Activities such as walking, swimming, cycling, and yoga are excellent starting points. These exercises help improve cardiovascular health, flexibility, and strength without putting undue stress on the SI joints.

- *Walking*: Begin with short walks around your neighborhood or on a treadmill. Gradually increase the duration and pace as you build endurance.
- *Swimming*: Water exercises are particularly beneficial as they provide resistance without impact, helping to strengthen muscles while minimizing joint stress.
- *Cycling*: Use a stationary bike or venture outdoors. Cycling is a great way to build leg strength and improve cardiovascular health.
- *Yoga and Stretching*: Incorporate gentle yoga poses and stretches to enhance flexibility, balance, and core strength. Poses like the child's pose, cat-cow stretch, and gentle spinal twists can be especially helpful.

3. **Gradually Increase Intensity and Duration:**

   As you become more fit and comfortable with your exercise routine, gradually increase the intensity and duration. This progressive approach allows your body to adapt and build strength over time.

   - *Strength Training*: Incorporate light weights or resistance bands to perform strength training exercises. Focus on major muscle groups, including the core, back, hips, and legs. Exercises such as squats, lunges, and bridges can help stabilize and support the SI joint.
   - *Cardiovascular Workouts*: Extend your cardio sessions by a few minutes each week. Aim for at least 150 minutes of moderate-intensity aerobic activity or 75 minutes of vigorous-intensity activity per week, as recommended by health guidelines.
   - *Flexibility and Balance*: Continue to work on flexibility and balance through yoga, Pilates, or targeted stretches. Improving these aspects can help prevent falls and maintain joint health.

4. **Listen to Your Body:**

   Pay close attention to how your body responds to exercise. While it's normal to experience some muscle soreness after a workout, sharp or persistent pain is a signal to stop and reevaluate your routine.

Ignoring such pain could lead to serious injuries. Adjust the intensity of your workouts, try different activities that might be less strenuous, or consult a healthcare professional for personalized advice if needed. Remember, your body knows best, and it's important to respect its signals.

5. **Stay Consistent and Motivated:**

Consistency is key to reaping the full benefits of regular exercise. Set realistic and achievable goals, and keep track of your progress to stay motivated. Find activities you genuinely enjoy, as this will make it easier to stick with your fitness routine in the long term.

Consider joining a class or finding a workout buddy to make exercising more enjoyable and to hold each other accountable. Staying motivated can sometimes be challenging, but finding the right support system and activities that bring you joy will help you stay on track.

By incorporating regular physical activity into your routine, you can significantly improve your quality of life and manage SI joint pain more effectively. Start slowly, listen to your body, and enjoy the journey towards better health and well-being.

Foods to Avoid for Sacroiliac Joint Pain

Certain foods are known to be highly inflammatory and should be avoided to help manage sacroiliac (SI) joint pain. These include:

- *Alcohol*: Can contribute to inflammation and dehydration, exacerbating joint pain.
- *Artificial Trans Fats*: Found in many processed foods, these fats can increase inflammation.
- *Dairy*: May cause inflammation in some individuals.
- *Processed Meats*: High in unhealthy fats and preservatives, which can promote inflammation.
- *Refined Carbohydrates*: Such as white bread and pastries, can spike blood sugar levels and increase inflammation.
- *Sugar*: Excessive consumption can lead to inflammation and weight gain.
- *Vegetable and Seed Oils*: High in omega-6 fatty acids, which can promote inflammation when consumed in excess.

By limiting or avoiding these foods, individuals with SI joint pain can potentially reduce inflammation and manage their symptoms more effectively.

Foods to Eat

Here are some anti-inflammatory foods that can greatly benefit someone experiencing SI joint pain:

1. **Fruits and Vegetables**
    - *Berries*: Blueberries, strawberries, raspberries, and blackberries are rich in antioxidants.
    - *Leafy Greens*: Spinach, kale, and Swiss chard contain powerful anti-inflammatory compounds.
    - *Tomatoes*: Packed with lycopene, which has anti-inflammatory properties.
2. **Healthy Fats**
    - *Olive Oil*: Extra virgin olive oil contains oleocanthal, an anti-inflammatory compound.
    - *Avocados*: Rich in healthy fats and antioxidants.
    - *Nuts and Seeds*: Walnuts, almonds, flaxseeds, and chia seeds provide omega-3 fatty acids.
3. **Fish**
    - *Fatty Fish*: Salmon, mackerel, sardines, and trout are high in omega-3 fatty acids that reduce inflammation.
4. **Whole Grains**
    - *Oats*: A good source of fiber and antioxidants.
    - *Brown Rice*: Contains healthy fiber and magnesium.
5. **Spices and Herbs**
    - *Turmeric*: Contains curcumin, a strong anti-inflammatory agent.
    - *Ginger*: Has gingerol, which reduces inflammation.

6. **Beverages**
    - ***Green Tea***: Contains catechins, which have anti-inflammatory effects.
7. **Legumes**
    - ***Beans***: Black beans, lentils, and chickpeas are excellent sources of fiber and protein.

Incorporating these foods into your diet can help manage and alleviate SI joint pain.

Sample Recipes

We understand that changing your diet can be challenging, especially when you are dealing with chronic pain. That's why we have put together some simple and delicious recipes that incorporate anti-inflammatory foods to help you get started:

Apple and Onion Soup

Ingredients:

- 3 organic apples, diced
- 2 medium yellow onions, sliced
- 6 cups vegetable broth
- 1 small leek, chopped
- 1 tbsp. avocado oil
- 1/2 tbsp. fresh rosemary, chopped
- 1/2 tbsp. fresh thyme

Instructions:

1. In a soup pot, heat avocado oil over medium heat.
2. Add diced apples and sliced onions to the pot and cook for 5-7 minutes until softened.
3. Stir in chopped leeks, rosemary, and thyme, and continue cooking for an additional 5 minutes.
4. Pour in vegetable broth and bring to a boil.
5. Reduce heat to low and let simmer for 20-25 minutes until flavors have developed.
6. Use an immersion blender or transfer soup into a blender to puree until smooth.
7. Serve hot with a sprinkle of fresh herbs on top if desired.

Trout Scrambler

Ingredients:

- 1 small potato, cut into 8 wedges
- 1/2 tsp. extra-virgin olive oil
- freshly ground black pepper, to taste
- 1 cup spinach
- 1 egg, scrambled
- 3 oz. trout filet
- dash of salt

Instructions:

1. Preheat the oven to 400°F.
2. Toss potato wedges with olive oil and black pepper in a baking dish.
3. Roast for 25 minutes until golden brown and tender.
4. In a separate pan, sauté spinach over medium heat until wilted.
5. Season trout filet with salt and cook in the same pan as the spinach for about 3-4 minutes on each side or until cooked through.
6. Meanwhile, scramble an egg in a small pan over low heat.

7. Assemble by placing roasted potatoes on a plate, followed by sautéed spinach, scrambled egg, and finally the cooked trout filet.
8. Serve hot for a filling and nutritious breakfast or brunch option.

Grilled Halibut Niçoise with Mixed Vegetables

Ingredients:

- 4 pcs. large eggs
- 1-1/2 lb. halibut filets, skin on
- 1/4 cup plus 2 tbsp. canola oil
- salt
- pepper
- 2 lbs. mixed vegetables in season, like romano beans, scallions, new potatoes, halved small eggplants, and garlic flower buds
- 4 cups red leaf, butter, or romaine lettuce, torn
- 1 cup tomatoes, halved
- 1 bunch small breakfast radishes, trimmed and halved lengthwise
- 1 cup green olive tapenade

Instructions:

1. Boil water. Add the eggs and cook for about 7 minutes.
2. Put the eggs in ice water to cool.
3. Put the grill on medium-high heat.
4. Use 2 tablespoons of the oil to rub on the halibut.
5. Season the filets with salt and pepper according to taste.
6. Put the filets, skin side down, on the grill.

7. Grill for between 5 to 8 minutes or until the skin is charred and the filets are cooked through.
8. Turn the filets and continue cooking for a minute more.
9. Remove the filets from the grill and put them on a plate.
10. Take the charred skin out. Set the fish aside.
11. In a large bowl, toss the mixed vegetables in the remaining canola oil. Add salt and pepper to season.
12. Grill the vegetables. Turn occasionally. The vegetables will be cooked at different times.
13. Transfer the vegetables to a plate when they are done, tender, and a bit charred.
14. Peel and halve the eggs.
15. Put the halibut filets, radishes, tomatoes, eggs, and grilled vegetables on a bed of lettuce leaves.
16. Drizzle green olive tapenade over the fish and vegetables.
17. Serve some of the tapenade on the side.

Salmon Fry

Ingredients:

- salmon
- 1/2 tsp. smoked paprika
- 1/2 tsp. garlic powder

Instructions:

1. Cut salmon into small filets.
2. Combine smoked paprika and garlic powder in a bowl.
3. Rub the mixture onto both sides of the salmon filets.
4. Heat a non-stick pan over medium heat.
5. Add a drizzle of oil to the pan.
6. Once the pan is hot, add salmon filets to the pan, skin side down.
7. Cook for 5-6 minutes on each side or until the fish is cooked through and flakes easily with a fork.
8. Remove from heat and let cool for a few minutes before serving.
9. Serve with your choice of sides, such as roasted vegetables or rice.

Kale Salad with Strawberry & Almonds

Ingredients:

- 1 bunch of kale
- 1/2 cup sliced strawberries
- 1/4 cup sliced almonds
- 1 lemon pulp juice
- 1/8 tsp. salt
- 1/8 tsp. black pepper
- 1 tbsp. agave
- 2 tbsp. of olive oil

Instructions:

1. Wash and dry the kale leaves, then remove the tough stems.
2. Tear or chop the leaves into small pieces and place in a mixing bowl.
3. In a separate bowl, whisk together lemon juice, agave, olive oil, salt, and pepper until well combined.
4. Pour dressing over the kale and use your hands to massage it into the leaves for about 2 minutes.
5. This will help to soften the leaves and make them easier to eat.
6. Add sliced strawberries and almonds to the kale mixture, and toss until evenly distributed.
7. Serve as a refreshing side dish or add a protein such as grilled chicken or tofu to make it a complete meal.

Tuna Salad

Ingredients:

- 1/2 cup pecans
- 1 cup chicken breast, steamed and cubed
- 1 cup tuna in oil
- salt, and pepper to taste

Instructions:

1. Preheat the oven to 350°F (175°C).
2. Spread pecans on a baking sheet and bake for about 10 minutes, until lightly toasted.
3. In a mixing bowl, combine the chicken breast, tuna, salt, and pepper.
4. Mix well until all ingredients are evenly distributed.
5. Once the pecans are cooled, chop them into small pieces and add them to the mixture.
6. Serve as a sandwich filling or as a topping for salads or crackers for a protein-packed snack.

Orange-Walnut Salad

Ingredients:

- 2 cups romaine lettuce, chopped coarsely
- 1 cucumber, peeled and deseeded, quartered lengthwise and chopped
- 1 cup arugula
- 2 navel oranges, peeled and chopped
- 1/4 cup red onion, sliced thinly
- 1 tbsp. walnut oil
- 2 tbsp. walnuts, chopped
- 1 tbsp. red wine vinegar
- 2 oz. blue cheese, gluten-free

Instructions:

1. In a large bowl, combine romaine lettuce, cucumber, arugula, oranges, and red onion.
2. Drizzle with walnut oil and toss to evenly coat the salad ingredients.
3. Add in chopped walnuts and crumbled blue cheese.
4. In a small bowl, whisk together red wine vinegar and a pinch of salt and pepper.
5. Pour dressing over the salad and toss until all ingredients are well combined.
6. Serve as a light lunch or side dish for a flavorful burst of citrus and nutty flavors.

Strawberry, Blueberry, and Spinach Salad

Ingredients:

- 5 strawberries, chopped
- 10 blueberries, chopped
- 1-1/2 cups baby spinach
- 1 oz. crumbled goat cheese
- 4 walnuts, crushed

For the salad dressing:

- 1/2 tbsp. extra-virgin olive oil
- cracked black pepper
- 1/2 tbsp. rice wine vinegar

Instructions:

1. In a large bowl, combine chopped strawberries, blueberries, and baby spinach.
2. Crumble goat cheese on top of the salad mixture.
3. In a small bowl, whisk together olive oil, cracked black pepper, and rice wine vinegar to create the dressing.
4. Drizzle the dressing over the salad and toss until all ingredients are evenly coated.

5. Top with crushed walnuts for an added crunch and nutty flavor.
6. Enjoy as a refreshing side dish or light meal option packed with antioxidants and healthy fats from the walnuts.

Kale Fried Rice

Ingredients:

- 2 tbsp. coconut oil
- 2 whole eggs
- 2 large garlic cloves, minced
- 3 large green onions, thinly sliced
- 1 cup of carrots, cut into matchsticks
- 1 cup of Brussels sprouts, diced
- 1 medium bunch of kale, ribs removed, and the leaves shredded
- 2 cups brown rice, cooked and cooled
- 1/4 tsp. Himalayan salt
- 1/4 cup of lemon balm leaves, diced
- 3/4 cups of shredded coconut, unsweetened variety
- fresh cilantro, for garnishing

Instructions:

1. Heat up a teaspoon of oil in a large skillet over medium-high heat.
2. Pour in the egg mixture.
3. Cook the eggs while occasionally stirring.
4. Remove from the pan and set aside.
5. Pour another teaspoon of coconut oil into the pan, along with Brussels sprouts, carrots, garlic, and green onions.
6. Occasionally stir until the vegetables become tender.

7. Add kale and salt.
8. Remove from the pan and put them into where the egg is.
9. Put the remaining coconut oil into the pan. Add in coconut flakes, stirring frequently
10. Add rice and stir it in.
11. Add the egg and vegetable mixture to the pan, as well as the lemon balm leaves.
12. Stir to combine and heat through.
13. Transfer to a serving bowl and garnish with fresh cilantro.
14. Serve and enjoy.

Instant Pot Bone Broth

Ingredients:

- 1 instant pot
- 4 whole celeries, ribbed
- 3 whole carrots, halved
- 1 onion, sliced in half
- 3 to 4 lb. grass-fed beef bones, roasted
- 1 bay leaf
- 2 cloves garlic, crushed with a knife
- 1 tbsp. apple cider vinegar
- 1 tsp. Himalayan pink salt

Instructions:

1. Put the beef bones on a baking sheet made of glass and season as desired with a sprinkle of salt.
2. Place the bones in an oven preheated to 420°F and let them roast for 30 minutes.
3. Flip them over and leave them for another 20 minutes.
4. Place the ingredients in the instant pot. Add the bones first, then followed by the remaining vegetables and seasoning.
5. Pour in clean water until it reaches an inch below the instant pot's max fill line.
6. Seal the instant pot and leave it on manual high pressure for approximately 75 minutes.

7. Remove both the vegetables and bones. Filter the broth using a fine-mesh strainer.
8. Pour the broth back into the instant pot.
9. You may use it immediately as a soup base or let it cool before storing it in the freezer for future use.

Garlic Hummus

Ingredients:

- 12 heads of garlic, roasted
- 2 tsp. virgin coconut oil
- 2 12-cup muffin tins
- extra trays of ice cube

Instructions:

1. Preheat the oven to 400°F.
2. Cut off the top of each garlic head to make the top of the cloves visible.
3. Put each garlic head in a muffin tin cup.
4. Rub the top of the garlic heads with coconut oil.
5. Use the second muffin tin to cover the first one.
6. Put in the oven and wait for 30 minutes to bake.
7. Take the garlic cloves out of the heads.
8. You may place 4-5 cloves of garlic in each ice cube tray section to store leftovers.
9. Use olive oil to cover cloves and freeze.
10. Squeeze the frozen roasted garlic cubes out of the trays and store them using a container.

Blueberry Pancakes with Whipped Cream

Ingredients:

- 2 organic eggs
- 1 tbsp. of coconut oil or melted butter
- 1/2 tsp vanilla
- 1 tbsp. xylitol
- 1/2 cup almond flour, add 1 tbsp. for thicker pancakes
- 1/2 cup tapioca flour
- 1/4 cup light coconut milk
- salt, to taste

For toppings:

- 1/2 cup fresh blueberries
- whipped cream
- Optional: pecans and cinnamon

Instructions:

1. In a blender, blend the eggs and coconut oil/butter together.
2. Add vanilla extract and xylitol to the egg mixture.
3. In a separate bowl, combine almond flour, tapioca flour, and salt.
4. Slowly add the dry ingredients into the blender while blending until smooth.
5. Pour in light coconut milk and blend once more for about 15 seconds.

6. Heat up a skillet over medium heat with 1 tbsp of coconut oil or butter.
7. Use a 1/4 cup measuring cup to pour the batter onto the skillet for each pancake.
8. Cook for about 3 minutes on one side, or until small bubbles appear.
9. Flip the pancake and cook for an additional 2-3 minutes.
10. Repeat with the remaining batter.
11. Serve pancakes hot with fresh blueberries and a dollop of whipped cream on top.
12. For an extra crunch, add some chopped pecans and sprinkle cinnamon over the whipped cream.

Energy Oats

Ingredients:

- 1 cup rolled oats
- 1 tbsp. walnuts
- 1 tbsp. flaxseed
- 1 tbsp. almonds, sliced
- 1 cup blueberries or fruit of choice
- 1 cup almond or soy milk

Instructions:

1. In a jar or container, combine oats, walnuts, flaxseed, and almonds.
2. Add in blueberries or fruit of choice.
3. Pour almond or soy milk over the mixture.
4. Mix well and cover the jar/container with a lid.
5. Place in the refrigerator for at least an hour, but preferably overnight.
6. In the morning, simply grab your jar/container and enjoy the cold or heat up in the microwave for a warm breakfast option.
7. For added sweetness, drizzle honey or maple syrup on top before serving.

Tomato and Basil Soup

Ingredients:

- 1 medium-sized onion, chopped
- 1 clove garlic, sliced finely
- 2 tablespoons olive oil
- 3 pcs. vine tomatoes or 8 pcs. cherry tomatoes, chopped
- 400 g can plum tomatoes
- 150 ml water
- 5 leaves of fresh basil or 1 tsp. dried basil
- 1 tsp. salt
- pepper

Instructions:

1. In a large pot, heat olive oil over medium-high heat.
2. Add chopped onions and sauté until translucent.
3. Stir in sliced garlic and cook for an additional minute.
4. Add in chopped vine or cherry tomatoes and cook for 5 minutes, stirring occasionally.
5. Pour in canned plum tomatoes, including the juices, and bring to a boil.
6. Reduce heat to low and simmer for 15 minutes.
7. Using an immersion blender or regular blender, puree the soup until smooth.

8. Return soup to pot if using a regular blender and add water, fresh or dried basil, salt, and pepper.
9. Cook for an additional 5 minutes on low heat.
10. Serve hot and garnish with additional basil leaves if desired.

Roasted Broccoli and Salmon

Ingredients:

- 1-1/2 lbs. or 1 bunch broccoli, cut into florets
- 4 tbsp. avocado oil, divided
- 1 tsp salt
- 1 tsp pepper
- 4 pcs. salmon filets, deskinned
- 1 pc. jalapeño or red Fresno chile deseeded and sliced into thin rings
- 2 tbsp. unseasoned rice vinegar
- 2 tbsp. capers drained

Instructions:

1. Preheat the oven to 425°F (220°C).
2. In a large bowl, toss broccoli florets with 3 tablespoons of avocado oil, salt, and pepper.
3. Spread the seasoned broccoli evenly on a baking sheet and roast for 20-25 minutes or until tender.
4. While the broccoli is roasting, season salmon filets with remaining avocado oil, salt, and pepper.
5. After the broccoli has cooked for 10 minutes, place the salmon filets on top of the vegetables on the baking sheet.
6. Sprinkle sliced jalapeño or red Fresno chile over the salmon and return to the oven.

7. Roast for an additional 12-15 minutes or until salmon is cooked through and flakes easily with a fork.
8. In a small bowl, mix together rice vinegar and capers.
9. Drizzle over the roasted broccoli and salmon before serving.
10. Serve hot and enjoy this delicious and healthy dish!

Tuna and Veggies Wrap

Ingredients:

- 2 pcs. whole-grain tortillas
- 1 cup cucumber, sliced
- 1 tbsp. low-fat Italian dressing
- 1 cup carrots, julienned

Instructions:

1. Lay out the tortillas on a flat surface.
2. In a small bowl, toss cucumber slices with Italian dressing until evenly coated.
3. Place half of the cucumbers in the center of each tortilla.
4. Top with julienned carrots.
5. Add tuna on top of the vegetables.
6. Roll up the tortillas tightly and secure them with toothpicks if needed.
7. Serve as is or lightly grill for 2-3 minutes to make it warm and crispy on the outside.

Enjoy this nutritious and flavorful wrap filled with veggies and protein from tuna!

Barley and Chicken Soup

Ingredients:

- 4 cups vegetable broth
- 4 cups chicken broth
- 2-1/2 lb. chicken breast, bone and skin removed, cubed
- 2 cups butternut squash, peeled and cubed
- 2 cups yellow summer squash
- 2 cups cubed zucchini squash
- 1 cup white onion, diced
- 1 cup broccoli florets
- 8 oz. fresh mushrooms, chopped
- 1 cup barley
- 2 cups water
- 1 tbsp. garlic, minced
- 1 whole bay leaf
- 1/4 tsp. sea salt
- 1/4 tsp. ground black pepper

Instructions:

1. Pour the water, vegetable broth, and chicken broth into a large pot.
2. Add the chicken cubes, onion, garlic, bay leaf, salt, and black pepper.
3. Using medium-high heat, bring the contents of the pot to a boil.
4. Reduce the heat to low. Simmer for an hour.

5. Add the barley, broccoli, butternut squash, yellow summer squash, zucchini, and mushrooms into the pot.
6. Bring back to a boil.
7. Lower it to a simmer for about 60 to 120 minutes, or until vegetables have achieved your desired texture.
8. Transfer into a serving bowl immediately.

Garlic-Cashews Red Pasta

Ingredients:

- 1 lb. pasta
- 1/2 cup cashews, ground into a powder
- 1/2 cup vegan cream cheese
- 1/4 cup extra-virgin olive oil (reserve for drizzling)
- 1 tbsp. tomato paste, optional
- 1 red bell pepper
- 4 cloves garlic
- black pepper, to taste
- salt, to taste

Instructions:

1. Cook the pasta according to package instructions.
2. In a blender, blend together the red bell pepper, garlic cloves, cashew powder, vegan cream cheese, and tomato paste (if using) until smooth.
3. Heat the olive oil in a large pan over medium heat.
4. Add the blended sauce to the pan and cook for about 5 minutes, stirring occasionally.
5. Drain the cooked pasta and add it to the sauce in the pan.
6. Stir everything together until well combined.
7. Season with salt and black pepper to taste.
8. Serve hot and drizzle with extra olive oil if desired.

Exotic Empanadas

Ingredients:

- 3 ox. lean ground beef
- 3 oz. mushrooms, chopped
- 1/4 cup onion, chopped finely
- 2 tsp. garlic, chopped finely
- 1/2 cup tomatoes, chopped
- 1/4 tsp. paprika
- 6 green olives, chopped
- 1/4 tsp. ground cumin
- 1/8 tsp. ground cinnamon
- 8 square gyoza wrappers
- 1 large egg, beaten
- 1 tbsp. olive oil

Instructions:

1. In a large pan, heat olive oil over medium-high heat.
2. Add the chopped onions and garlic, cooking until fragrant.
3. Add in the ground beef and cook until browned.
4. Stir in the chopped mushrooms, tomatoes, paprika, cumin, and cinnamon.
5. Cook for an additional 5 minutes or until vegetables are soft.
6. Remove from heat and let cool for a few minutes.
7. Preheat the oven to 375°F (190°C).

8. On a clean surface, lay out your gyoza wrappers.
9. Spoon about 1 tablespoon of the beef mixture into the center of each wrapper.
10. Add a small amount of chopped green olives on top of the beef mixture.
11. Brush egg wash around the edges of the wrapper and fold in half, pressing down to seal.
12. Use a fork to crimp along the edges for a decorative touch.
13. Place empanadas on a baking sheet lined with parchment paper.
14. Brush tops with remaining egg wash for a golden crust.
15. Bake for 15-20 minutes or until edges are lightly browned.
16. Serve hot and enjoy!

Pork Tenderloin

Ingredients:

- 1 lb. pork tenderloin
- pepper
- salt
- 1 tbsp. coconut oil

Instructions:

1. Preheat the oven to 400°F (200°C).
2. Season the pork tenderloin with salt and pepper on all sides.
3. In a large skillet, heat coconut oil over medium-high heat.
4. Once hot, add the seasoned pork tenderloin to the skillet.
5. Sear each side for about 2-3 minutes or until browned.
6. Transfer the tenderloin to a baking dish and place it in the oven for 15-20 minutes or until the internal temperature reaches 145°F (63°C).
7. Let the pork rest for 5-10 minutes before slicing and serving.
8. Enjoy with your favorite side dishes, such as roasted vegetables or mashed potatoes.

Baked Turkey Wings

Ingredients:

- 4 pcs. or about 5 lbs. whole turkey wings
- 1 tbsp olive oil
- salt and pepper
- 1 tsp paprika

Instructions:

1. Preheat the oven to 375°F (190°C).
2. Rinse and pat dry the turkey wings.
3. Rub olive oil all over the wings and season generously with salt, pepper, and paprika.
4. Place the wings on a baking sheet lined with foil or parchment paper.
5. Bake for 45-50 minutes or until golden brown and fully cooked (internal temperature should reach 165°F/74°C).
6. Let the wings rest for a few minutes before serving.
7. Serve hot as an appetizer or main dish with your choice of dipping sauce. Enjoy!

Conclusion

As you reach the end of this guide on Sacroiliac Joint Disease management, it's important to recognize and celebrate your commitment to understanding and improving your health. Your journey through this guide shows a proactive approach to managing your condition and enhancing your quality of life. By focusing on various strategies for managing Sacroiliac Joint Disease, you've equipped yourself with valuable knowledge that can make a significant difference.

Sacroiliac Joint Disease can present many challenges, but you've learned that an integrated management plan can lead to meaningful improvements. Managing this condition requires a multifaceted approach, including diet, exercise, lifestyle changes, and medical interventions. Each of these elements plays a vital role in reducing pain and improving function.

One effective way to manage Sacroiliac Joint Disease is through dietary adjustments. The food you eat impacts inflammation levels and overall joint health. By including anti-inflammatory foods such as fruits, vegetables, lean proteins, and healthy fats in your diet, you can help reduce inflammation and alleviate symptoms.

These dietary choices not only reduce pain but also promote general well-being. Understanding the relationship between diet and joint health empowers you to make informed decisions. Foods rich in antioxidants protect your cells, while fiber-rich options support digestive health, which is linked to inflammation and immune function. This holistic approach ensures that you're not just treating symptoms but creating a healthier internal environment.

Hydration is another crucial component of managing Sacroiliac Joint Disease. Adequate water intake helps maintain joint lubrication and supports various bodily functions. Herbal teas and broths can offer additional anti-inflammatory benefits.

In addition to dietary changes, staying active with regular exercise is essential. Low-impact exercises such as swimming, walking, or yoga can strengthen the muscles around your sacroiliac joint, providing better support and reducing strain. Physical activity enhances mobility and contributes to overall health, making it a key aspect of your management plan.

Managing Sacroiliac Joint Disease is an ongoing journey. There will be days when sticking to your plan feels challenging. During these times, remember the long-term benefits you're working towards reduced pain, increased mobility, and an improved sense of well-being. Keeping a journal to track your progress and note any changes in your symptoms can provide valuable insights and motivation.

Consulting healthcare professionals such as physical therapists, nutritionists, or dietitians can offer personalized guidance tailored to your needs. Their expertise can help you navigate challenges and create a balanced management plan that supports both your joints and overall health. Their support can make your journey more manageable and sustainable.

Lifestyle factors such as adequate sleep and stress management also play a significant role in managing Sacroiliac Joint Disease. Ensuring you get enough restful sleep helps your body repair and recover, while stress management techniques like meditation or deep breathing exercises can reduce muscle tension and pain. Combining these practices with your dietary and exercise efforts creates a well-rounded approach to managing your condition.

As you continue on this path, it's important to listen to your body. Pay attention to how different strategies affect your symptoms and adjust your plan accordingly. Each person's response to management techniques can vary, so being mindful and patient with yourself is crucial in finding what works best for you.

Thank you for dedicating your time and effort to exploring this guide on Sacroiliac Joint Disease management. Your willingness to learn and adapt is commendable and will lead to positive outcomes. Stay proactive, seek support when needed, and prioritize your health. Your commitment to positive changes sets a foundation for long-term wellness and a more comfortable, active life.

This journey is about more than managing a condition; it's about embracing a healthier lifestyle. Your dedication to effective management strategies lays the groundwork for sustained well-being. Remember, each step you take towards managing your condition is a step towards a brighter future. By focusing on what you can control and staying informed, you're paving the way for a more comfortable and active life.

In conclusion, managing Sacroiliac Joint Disease requires a comprehensive and proactive approach. By combining dietary adjustments, regular exercise, adequate hydration, and lifestyle changes, you can significantly reduce your symptoms and improve your quality of life. Your journey doesn't end here; it's an ongoing process of making mindful choices and seeking continuous improvement. Stay dedicated, and know that every positive change brings you closer to a healthier, more vibrant you.

FAQs for Sacroiliac Joint Disease Management Through Diet

What foods should I avoid to manage Sacroiliac Joint Disease?

To reduce inflammation, it's best to avoid processed foods, refined sugars, trans fats, and red meats. These can contribute to inflammation and exacerbate symptoms.

What are the best foods to eat for reducing inflammation in Sacroiliac Joint Disease?

Anti-inflammatory foods include fruits, vegetables, whole grains, lean proteins (such as fish and poultry), nuts, seeds, and healthy fats like olive oil and avocado. Omega-3 fatty acids found in fish like salmon and flaxseeds are particularly beneficial.

Can an anti-inflammatory diet completely cure Sacroiliac Joint Disease?

While an anti-inflammatory diet can significantly reduce symptoms by lowering inflammation, it is not a cure for SIJD. It should be part of a comprehensive treatment plan that may include physical therapy, medications, and other interventions.

How quickly can I expect to see results from dietary changes?

The timeline for seeing improvements varies from person to person. Some individuals may notice reduced pain and inflammation within a few weeks, while others might take a few months to experience significant benefits.

Are there any specific dietary supplements that can help with Sacroiliac Joint Disease?

Certain supplements, such as omega-3 fatty acids, turmeric (curcumin), and glucosamine, may help reduce inflammation and support joint health. Always consult with a healthcare provider before starting any new supplement regimen.

Is it necessary to eliminate all dairy and gluten from my diet?

Not necessarily. While some people with SIJD find relief by avoiding dairy and gluten, it's not required for everyone. It's advisable to try eliminating these foods and monitor how your body responds, then reintroduce them to see if symptoms worsen.

How can I ensure I'm getting all the necessary nutrients on an anti-inflammatory diet?

Focus on eating a balanced variety of whole foods to cover your nutritional bases. If you're concerned about potential deficiencies, consider consulting a nutritionist or dietitian who can help you create a meal plan that meets all your nutritional needs while managing inflammation.

References and Helpful Links

7 home remedies for sacroiliac joint pain. (n.d.). https://www.alethahealth.com/post/home-remedies-for-sacroiliac-joint-pain

Clinic, C. (2024c, April 30). 10 foods that help ease your arthritis pain. Cleveland Clinic. https://health.clevelandclinic.org/top-10-foods-power-ease-arthritis-pain

Harvard Health. (2024, March 26). Foods that fight inflammation. https://www.health.harvard.edu/staying-healthy/foods-that-fight-inflammation

Admin. (2020, October 27). The best foods for Healthy joints | Inflammatory foods to avoid. VOSCT. https://vosct.com/best-foods-for-healthy-joints/

George, M., MD. (n.d.). All about sacroiliitis. Spine-health. https://www.spine-health.com/conditions/sacroiliac-joint-dysfunction/all-about-sacroiliitis

Mph, S. B. M. (n.d.). Anti-Inflammatory foods to try for neck pain. Spine-health. https://www.spine-health.com/conditions/neck-pain/anti-inflammatory-foods-try-neck-pain

Faco, S. Y. D. (n.d.). Sacroiliac joint dysfunction (SI joint pain). Spine-health. https://www.spine-health.com/conditions/sacroiliac-joint-dysfunction/sacroiliac-joint-dysfunction-si-joint-pain

Sacroiliac joint pain - aftercare: MedlinePlus Medical Encyclopedia. (n.d.). https://medlineplus.gov/ency/patientinstructions/000610.htm#:~:text=Your%20provider%20may%20recommend%20these,to%203%20times%20a%20day.

Kemp, W., MD. (n.d.). How your diet can affect your SI joint. Spine-health. https://www.spine-health.com/blog/how-your-diet-can-affect-your-si-joint

Elder, S., DC. (n.d.). Common triggers of SI joint pain and how to prevent a flare-up. Spine-health. https://www.spine-health.com/blog/common-triggers-si-joint-pain-and-how-prevent-flare-up#:~:text=Eat%20a%20healthy%2C%20anti%2Dinflammatory,and%20refined%20sugar%2C%20is%20beneficial.

www.ingramcontent.com/pod-product-compliance
Lightning Source LLC
LaVergne TN
LVHW012034060526
838201LV00061B/4593